T0129264

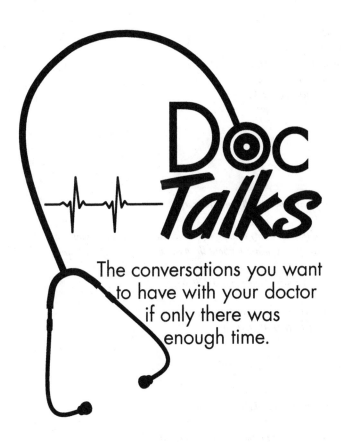

# Doc Talks

The conversations you want
to have with your doctor
if only there was
enough time.

Dr. Justin Abbott DO/MBA

authorHOUSE®

*AuthorHouse™*
*1663 Liberty Drive*
*Bloomington, IN 47403*
*www.authorhouse.com*
*Phone: 1 (800) 839-8640*

*Published by AuthorHouse   03/31/2016*

*ISBN: 978-1-5049-8731-8 (sc)*
*ISBN: 978-1-5049-8730-1 (e)*

*Print information available on the last page.*

# CONTENTS

Chapter 1 Hypertension, The Silent Killer.................1

Chapter 2 Hyperlipidemia (High Cholesterol)...........7

Chapter 3 Diabetes....................................12

Chapter 4 Adult Vaccination Guide .......................18

Chapter 5 Cancer Screening...................................22

Chapter 6 Alcohol .....................................26

Chapter 7 Tobacco .....................................32

Chapter 8 What you should know about your

            doctor .....................................39

# CHAPTER ONE

## Hypertension, The Silent Killer

## Medical Facts:

According to the CDC, seventy million Americans are currently diagnosed with high blood pressure. In medical jargon, we commonly call high blood pressure hypertension and we abbreviate it HTN. HTN is a disorder that is characterized by an elevated pressure of the flow of blood in your arteries all over your body. There can be many different causes of high blood pressure, and it can exist just by itself, we call this essential hypertension. Essential HTN is likely a genetic trait passed on to you from your parents. Many of the causes of HTN are reversible, and you should have this discussion this with your doctor. A few examples would be being overweight, sleep apnea, narrowing of the blood vessels to your kidneys, certain tumors, and certain behaviors such as excess stimulant intake (caffeine) and salt intake that can increase blood pressure.

High blood pressure typically does not have any symptoms associated with it, hence the term **the silent killer**, as it can be present and damaging your body for many years before you know you have it. At very high levels you can have nose bleeds or even sometimes headaches- this is usually associated with severe HTN. It is possible also to have a stroke due to high blood pressure, however this is usually associated with very extreme high blood pressure. Unfortunately the vast majority of us can walk along in life on a day to day basis and not know that our blood pressure is significantly elevated, which is why it can be so dangerous.

High blood pressure hurts and changes our bodies in several ways. I want to try and describe this to you for a better understanding. Our blood flows away from our heart in blood vessels called arteries, and it flows back to the heart in blood vessels called veins. The venous side of the body and its associated right side of the heart is typically a low pressure system. The arterial side coming from the left heart is a much higher pressure circuit. These arteries that carry the blood away from the heart have a muscular layer inside them, similar to the rest of the muscles in our body. When stress and tension (elevated pressure) is put on the arteries muscle layer it reacts and the muscle becomes larger, more thickened and unfortunately stiffer. While this muscle bulking is typically good for the rest of the muscles in our body, it is bad for the muscles in our arteries.

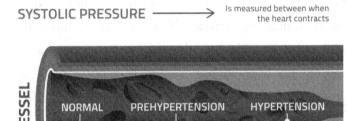

SYSTOLIC PRESSURE ⟶ Is measured between when the heart contracts

VESSEL

NORMAL    PREHYPERTENSION    HYPERTENSION

DIASTOLIC PRESSURE ⟶ Is measured between beats when the heart relaxes

**Blood Pressure**
VECTOR INFOGRAPHIC

Blood Pressure is the pressure exerted by circulating blood upon the walls of blood vessels.

Our arteries need to be dynamic, that is to be able to stretch and then relax as our heart beats in a pulsatile manner. The thicker the muscle layer in our arteries become the more stiff they become and, the less they can pulsate and they carry less blood. This is similar to thinking about a car tunnel with walls that grow inward, the thicker the walls grow inward, the less cars can fit through, in our case our blood molecules are the cars.

This decrease in ability to stretch combined with the increase in muscle growth in the artery and the increased pressure causes problems with the heart. Think of your heart as a pump at the bottom of a well. It pumps water up the well through a tube or hose like our heart pumps blood through our arteries. Now stand at the top of the well and squeeze the hose that the water is coming out of so only half of the liquid can get through it. What can you guess will happen with the pump? Over time the same things will happen with the heart, it will wear out. In the case of our heart instead of replacing pump seals and gaskets, we have to replace valves and give medicines. Our heart does not have the luxury of just being replaced, so it tries to compensate by making itself larger and more forceful. The heart dilates and builds up more muscle. Unfortunately, this is not a good thing, this reaction and compensation is what leads to the two different forms of congestive heart failure.

So the result of high blood pressure in the cardiovascular system is big muscled and stiff blood vessels as well as an enlarged heart. This process and attempt at compensation is what leads to heart disease (attacks and heart failure) as well as kidney disease and stroke. Below are x-rays showing how big the heart can become from hypertension. On the top is a normal chest x-ray and normal sized heart, and on the bottom is a heart that has congestive failure. Remember, this is about the only place in the body that bigger muscle is bad!

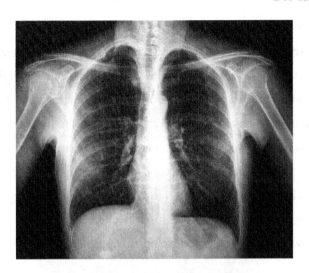

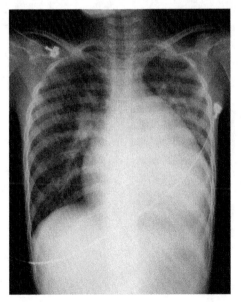

What is the answer? For a lot of Americans, diet modification and regular cardiac activity can be enough to lower your blood pressure. This is dependent on how high it is and other factors such as gender and race. For those of us where that is not enough, you need to have a talk with your doctor about which medications are right for you, the first step of course is just getting into the doctor and having it checked. We are incredibly lucky to have very well tolerated medicines with relatively few side effects at generic low costs. Talk to your doctor about which medicine may be right for you. And the biggest thing, get your blood pressure checked regularly so you know if and when you develop this problem.

# CHAPTER TWO

## Hyperlipidemia (High Cholesterol)

If you were ever to come into the hospital having a heart attack or stroke, once stabilized, one of the first things that your doctor will do is put you on a cholesterol medication. If you have heart disease or have had a stroke, it is arguably one of the most important medications for you to be taking.

The insides of our arteries have fatty sheets of deposits covering them that are made up of cholesterol. This is normal in all of us. This process starts at around 17 years old. Most of the fatty sheets are made up of a specific type of cholesterol called LDL cholesterol, short for low density lipoproteins. We get LDL cholesterol from food we eat and we make LDL cholesterol in our liver. Each of us are genetically programmed to make a certain amount of cholesterol so that if we are not eating sufficient, our bodies still have enough to function.

Some individuals have a genetic disorder where the liver makes a lot more LDL cholesterol than our body needs. Some of us eat all of the LDL we could ever need and unfortunately the liver makes it share anyways. The problem is, the more LDL cholesterol in your body and blood, the more plaques build up in your arteries. The more cholesterol you have in your arteries, the less blood that can fit through them- kind of like the same tunnel and car problem as in HTN. The less blood that can fit through, the more the muscle and tissue that the artery is supplying suffers and does not work well. This can happen in any artery in your body. It can happen in your legs and arms (peripheral vascular disease), intestines (ischemic bowel) or your heart (coronary artery disease and heart attacks) and your brain (stroke and microvascular disease).

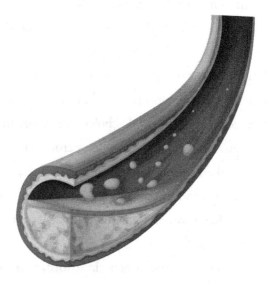

One of the big problems we can encounter is that every once in a while a LDL plaque becomes loose, and the blood carries it downstream until it becomes lodged and cannot move any further. This is kind of like a large rock rolling down a river, it can eventually act like a dam. When this happens in the arteries of the heart, you suffer a heart attack, in the brain, a stroke, and in the intestines, dead bowel.

What makes matters worse, this area that had the piece of cholesterol flake off is then exposed to blood flow at its base. The body recognizes this is an injury and tells our platelets to "repair" it. These platelets clump on each other and make a big ball of platelets over the "injury" forming a bigger blood clot. This ball of platelets gets so big that in can occlude the entire blood vessel where it happened causing more problems like the piece that went downstream in the artery. This then further causes heart muscle to die, brain tissue to die or bowel tissue to die depending on the location. Getting the body to not build up these LDL cholesterol plaques as well as controlling high blood pressure can prevent this whole process from happening.

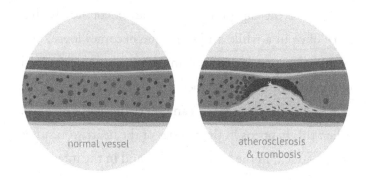

normal vessel

atherosclerosis
& trombosis

We have chemically studied the liver and now know how it makes cholesterol. We have found a specific enzyme that we can block with a medicine to cut down the process of building LDL cholesterol. In most cases, we can cut your LDL cholesterol in half, greatly decreasing the amount deposited in your arteries and hopefully preventing the problem in the first place.

Something we didn't expect to find with this medication is its ability to stabilize and concrete down plaques that already exist in arteries and make them more stable. This is why one of the first things your doctor does when you have a heart attack or stroke, is to put you on one of these medications; it acts like a glue to keep these plaques cemented down.

These medications, like all others have a few possible side effects that your doctor will talk to you about, they are typically quite minimal and most people tolerate these medicines very well. Thankfully, many are generic medications that are inexpensive to be on. What is most important is that you do not wait for an occurrence to happen before treating your high cholesterol. Get into your doctor and have your fasting cholesterol tested and talk about how often you should have it tested. Start making dietary changes now to help with this overall process, some red meats, cheeses, and creams are all high in cholesterol. Talk to your doctor about a lower fat low cholesterol diet.

Talk to your doctor also about the benefits of fish oils as a supplement as well as Coenzyme Q-10 that can sometimes be helpful in cholesterol management.

# CHAPTER THREE

## Diabetes

It all begins with the Pancreas. This fragile little organ sits behind the stomach and is very connected functionally to it. The pancreas produces several chemicals and hormones that aid in digestion and other processes, insulin is the one that is relevant to diabetes and arguably the most important. There are two historical types of Diabetes. **Type one** is where there is no insulin made by the pancreas, this disease typically manifests itself in the first two decades of life and requires complete insulin replacement. **Type two** diabetes is what is becoming an epidemic in this country and is largely behaviorally induced. The picture below shows some of the signs and symptoms of Type One diabetes, the signs and symptoms of Type Two can be much more subtle. Let me start by describing the process of insulin use and type two diabetes.

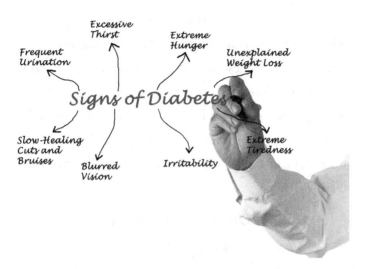

When you eat a donut, a big serving of rice or potatoes, or a candy bar or other largely carbohydrate (sugar) containing food, this stimulates the pancreas to make and release insulin to help clear this sugar from our bloodstream. It enables the sugar to get into the muscles and cells in our body to use it for energy. In our diet in America, we unfortunately eat too many of these carbohydrate rich foods. They are just too easily and cheaply available compared to other higher protein and more nutritious foods like fruits and vegetables and lean meats.

When we eat a donut or lots of bread or rolls or rice or potatoes, the pancreas then has to secrete an enormous amount of insulin to cover this food and clear the sugar out of the bloodstream and get it into cells that use it.

What happens in type II diabetes is that the pancreas either eventually runs out of its ability to make insulin, or the body becomes insensitive to all this insulin and it doesn't do its job anymore. The main job of insulin is to help sugar get out of the bloodstream and into cells to be used as energy. If insulin is lacking or ineffective, then sugar stays in the bloodstream and the cells effectively starve.

## IMPORTANCE OF INSULIN

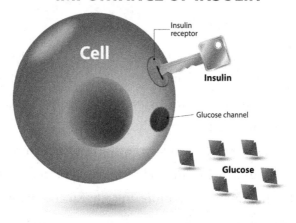

When these cells starve, they think it is because there is no sugar in the bloodstream, they do not know that indeed there really is sugar there, it just can't make it into the cell to use it. Think of insulin as the key to unlock the gate to let sugar get from the blood where it has no purpose, to the cell where it is used.

The muscle and brain cells and all of the cells of the body that can't access this sugar then release chemicals into the bloodstream to tell the liver to take its storage of sugar and release it so it can get the energy it needs. This makes the problem worse; it releases more sugar in the bloodstream that still cannot get into the cells where it is needed. This is the vicious cycle of type II diabetes.

The good news is that type 2 diabetes has many possible treatments both medically and with life habits. Some people, if diagnosed early enough, need no medicine at all and weight loss and regular exercise are sufficient treatment. For others, where this is not the case, we have great medicines to help your body become more sensitive to insulin and even help it make more if needed and able. Sometimes, further along in the disease usually after left undiagnosed for too long, insulin replacement shots can become necessary.

Diabetes, or rather the high sugars associated with it, cause many problems in the body. These elevated sugar levels in the bloodstream cause damage to the smallest blood vessels in the body. The kidneys, eyes, feet, heart and brain are all especially susceptible to the destructive effects of the elevated sugars of diabetes due to the small arteries and vessels in them. This is why having diabetes is a big risk factor for heart disease, strokes and kidney failure as well as vision problems. As seen in the picture below, diabetics also have an incredibly difficult time healing and tend to develop sores and ulcers, especially on their feet. This is why many diabetics have ended up with amputations in the past, they don't check their feet regularly, and it turns out, it is really important to do this.

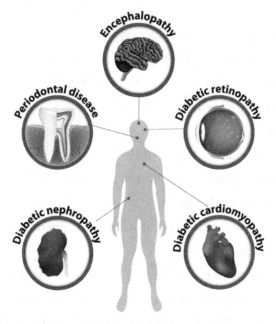

**DIABETES MELLITUS** *(Type 2)*

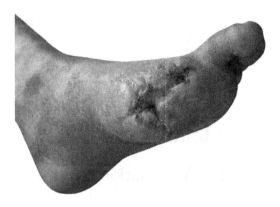

I recommend screening for diabetes once a year after age thirty unless you are overweight then you should start earlier and then yearly throughout life. Screening is accomplished in one of three possible ways; a fasting blood sugar which is part of most yearly physical tests, a sugar average test called a hemoglobin A1c that is available in most Family Practice offices, or by a sugar challenge test where you drink a specific sugar beverage and then test sugars hourly after that for a few hours. Please talk to your doctor at your next yearly physical about which test should be done on you as well as your family history and specific risk level. For diabetes, prevention is the best medicine. A diet with lots of lean proteins and meats and vegetables and regular cardiac exercise can go a long way towards prevention.

# CHAPTER FOUR

## Adult Vaccination Guide

**Shingles vaccine**: A good idea for essentially every one over sixty five and some select individuals maybe earlier. Shingles is a viral infection of the herpes family that causes a very painful rash on the skin. Having the vaccine can greatly reduce your chances of getting this illness. If you have already had this illness, I still recommend the vaccine as it can make you much less likely to have long term complications from this rash. Probably the number one complication I worry about from shingles infection is called Post- Herpetic Neuralgia (PHN). PHN is a condition where the virus continues to live in the nerves of the skin and the patient has chronic pain for sometimes the rest of his or her life on the skin in that area. Having this vaccine, greatly reduces the chance of PHN.

**Pneumonia vaccine**: Contrary to its name, this vaccine will not prevent you from getting routine run of the mill pneumonia!! What this vaccine does is protect you from getting the incredibly invasive infection of certain strains of the pneumonia bacteria that we know are more likely to be severe and fatal. Invasive Strep Pneumonia can be an illness requiring intensive care unit level of care. Unfortunately, pneumonia is the eighth highest cause of death in the United States annually and the number one cause of death by infection. This vaccine is targeted at these invasive strains that commonly cause death and go a long way to try and prevent them. This vaccine is especially important if you are chronically ill, smoke, or have chronic lung diseases.

**Whooping Cough/Tetanus/Diptheria (TDaP):** This vaccine has three components; the whooping cough component is in my opinion the most important, which is likely active and beneficial for 5-7 years, and the tetanus and diphtheria component which is likely active and good for a lot longer. The real importance with this vaccination is that immunity from whooping cough shots in childhood will wear off. In most cases of whooping cough outbreaks it is either those who have not been vaccinated or grandparents or parents whose immunity has worn off that are the ones who pass this disease on to others. It is a horrible illness with a cough that lasts one hundred days and is violent enough to break ribs in those who have it. For newborns, it unfortunately can be a fatal illness. Get updated on this vaccine as whooping cough is now occurring in outbreaks across our nation.

**Influenza vaccine**: This vaccine is aimed at the seasonal influenza virus that rotates around the world on a yearly basis. It changes slightly and we attempt to match our immunizations to what has gone through Asia the season prior as this is how it travels around the world. Historically these viruses can mutate and change and become more infective and more fatal such as the 1918 H1N1 Pandemic that killed 100 million people around the globe wiping out 3 percent of the earth's population. Influenza itself usually has a very abrupt onset with intense muscle aches and pains, fever well over one hundred degrees and a very dry non productive cough. Typically when you have this infection, you feel just shy of death and are pretty sure you have been run over by a train. It is horrific! It typically lasts 10 days with the worst of it being in the middle. It can be incredibly serious and is fatal for some, mostly the extremes of age or immune compromised. We do not have a good treatment for it and it is a miserable experience. We have done a great injustice to the word Flu. We use it commonplace to describe other viral infections calling them the "stomach flu" or a cold as "just a touch of the flu" in reality it is a distinct and much more serious illness. This vaccination is among the most important that exists in my opinion.

To those who have been made "sick" by the flu shot, that's not true! That is the vaccine working and tricking the body into thinking it is being infected. Your body has an awesomely intense immune system. The soreness and body aches and feeling miserable that some experience is just your immune system looking for and depositing immune complexes to kill the flu in tissues in your body! This passes in 24-48 hours. These folks that have this reaction are among those who actually have the best protection from the flu. There immune system has been fully sensitized and prepared.

**HPV- Human Papilloma Virus vaccination** is for young adolescents and adults. It protects against the virus that causes cervical cancer as well as Ano-genital cancer and cancers of the mouth. Both young men and women should receive these vaccines, as in men the infection can be without symptoms at all and they can then pass this infection on to other partners, men or women.

# CHAPTER FIVE

## Cancer Screening

## Males-

**Testicular cancer-** This cancer affects predominantly younger men who can be very healthy otherwise. This cancers peak incidence is between 15 and 35 years of age. Unless you are performing a testicular exam on yourself regularly, it can be growing and building for quite some time prior to manifesting itself through pain or swelling or otherwise. Make it a part of your physical with your doctor every year and have he or she show you what to look for on your own.

**Prostate cancer-** This type of cancer is in a round small walnut shaped gland that sits at the outlet of the bladder. There are many different types and levels of aggressiveness in this type of cancer. For ease, I break it up into two types or categories in my mind. The first is the kind that we are all going to get if we live long enough, a recent statistic I read somewhere state eighty percent of those over eighty years old will have a slow growing not incredibly invasive form of this cancer. The second type of cancer is the one I worry about missing as a primary care practitioner. It can set in earlier in life in the fourth and fifth decades and be much more aggressive and travel to other places in the body much faster than the other. It is important that if you start to develop any urinary symptoms such as inability to start a stream of urine, or a lot of frequency – having to go all the time, or not being able to empty the bladder all the way can be symptoms of this cancer and you should tell your doctor. There are two common ways to screen for this cancer. The first is physical palpation of the gland itself this is done rectally with the finger to actually feel the gland itself for any irregularities or large size. The second method is to draw a blood test for a marker in the blood related to the prostate gland, this has become quite controversial in recent times as certain groups feel it does more harm than good as it can be falsely elevated and lead to more testing than necessary. I feel we have unfortunately gotten away from the physical exam portion too much and rely on blood work that in some instances, misses a cancer. Talk to your doctor about both of these methods and if over forty, it should in my opinion be part of a physical exam yearly.

# Female cancer Screening

Breast cancer is being diagnosed much earlier and having much better success rates due to awareness and early intervention and screening. Women over forty should have a mammogram every year. Most women should have a physical yearly that includes a breast exam by their physician. If there is a family history of breast cancer in mother, sisters or Aunts I would start screening much earlier in life, talk to your doctor about specifics. Also, talk to your doctor about his/her perspective and advice on breast self-exams.

**Cervical cancer**- Screening for this type of cancer is quite important as usually by the time it has symptoms it can be advanced. A pap smear should be done in my opinion yearly for those over twenty one and then possibly spaced out to every three years based on specific risk level. Cervical cancer is caused by the HPV virus talked about in the vaccination chapter and can be almost entirely prevented by condom use and vaccination.

**Uterine cancer**- typically sets in later in life and the only sign sometimes can be monthly cycle changes. It is important to talk to your doctor about any cycle changes you experience as testing for this type of cancer can be done simultaneously when doing the pap smear by just sampling cells just inside the cervix.

**Ovarian cancer-** screening for this cancer is accomplished during the yearly exam. After the pap smear is obtained typically the sides of your uterus and the space where your ovaries sit are examined and felt to not have any masses or fullness on exam. There is a blood test for monitoring those that have ovarian cancer – but it is not good enough yet to be used to screen for cancer in the general population it lacks in sensitivity and specificity, but hopefully this will change in the very near future.

**Colon Cancer-** Both men and women should be screened for colon cancer. My recommendation is that all adults at age 50 have a colonoscopy. If there has been a family member with it diagnosed, then screening should start earlier. We know that there are certain types of growths that begin benign and then take several important steps over a certain period of years to turn into a cancer. We have figured out that most of these begin in the forties and turn into the cancer in the fifties and sixties. If we catch them before they make this change and remove them, it can save your life. Some changes in the bowel habits can lead to earlier screening. I typically consider it for most men or women who are having black tarry stools or any color of blood in their stool. Other things such as change in caliber of stool may also hasten this screening test. It is also a good idea every several years to have a rectal exam by your doctor in addition to fecal testing for blood.

# CHAPTER SIX

## Alcohol

To begin with, alcohol has a long history in this country, in fact it is tied very closely to certain recreations like barbecues, football games, yard work, boating, camping, hunting, and even generally just weekends. In moderation, like a glass of wine nightly, alcohol can just be a way to relax for some people and wind down for the day, and in this small quantity is typically not harmful to the body. In contrast, 2-3 glasses of wine every night can be quite harmful to your health. In a societal context, alcohol is a public health problem. According to the National Institutes of Health, 88,000 deaths occur in the US annually due to alcohol. Over 97,000 college students every year between the ages of 18-24 report alcohol related sexual assault or date rape every year. Alcohol is attributed to over 696,000 assaults every year in this same age group. The NIH has found that alcohol use directly increases the risk of mouth, esophageal, pharyngeal, laryngeal, and liver and breast cancer.

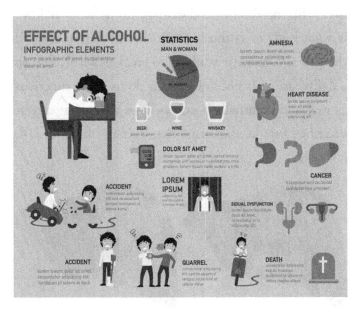

Alcohol is a toxic chemical in the body. It has to be broken down and detoxified by the liver. The liver does this with what we refer to as zero order kinetics, meaning that the liver can only detoxify a certain amount of alcohol per hour. Let's say for example your liver is capable of detoxifying one beer per hour. If you drink 2 beers it would take 2 hours to detoxify and get it out of your system, likewise if you were to drink a six pack, it would take 6 hours to get this amount of alcohol out of your system no matter how much time it took you to drink them. This is unlike other processes in our body where typically the more of something there is to break down the faster it can do it, this is not true for alcohol and the liver. This metabolism and damage from the breakdown is what leads to cirrhosis (destruction) of your liver. If the liver is constantly working to break down alcohol on a daily basis it is not available to do its other functions as well and eventually becomes filled with what can be described best as scar tissue that does not function like it should.

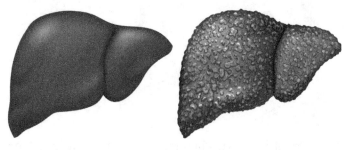

This is how chronic alcohol consumption can damage your liver. Unfortunately as well, the liver works in concert with the kidneys and failure of one can lead to failure of the other meaning if you destroy your liver with alcohol your kidneys will likely not be far behind. Also of concern is your heart, chronic alcohol consumption through similar processes in the liver cause the heart to dilate and stretch and can eventually lead to heart failure. Indirectly also through the sheer calorie consumption, it can lead to diabetes as typically most folks who chronically drink more than one or two drinks a day end up overweight with the typical "beer belly" the most medically harmful place to carry fat on your body.

In addition to my health concerns with alcohol, I also have grave concerns over its direct effects of intoxication. It does several things to your brain and we have all witnessed or heard of these effects in slang terms. For example, you have heard the term that she thought he was cute because she had beer goggles on- meaning her perception was altered. What about the phrase he or she is a "mean drunk" meaning a nice person until intoxicated and then turns mean.

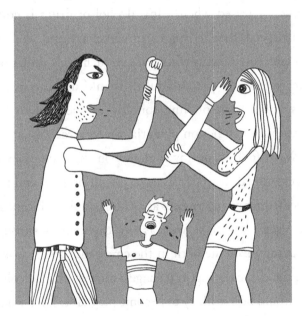

Or what about just the sheer number of excuses that can be attributed to being drunk, for example I was drunk I didn't mean to sleep with that person, or get in a car with that person. Or I didn't mean to beat up that person and go to jail. There are all sorts of behaviors that we associate with intoxication for a reason, it alters your decision making. This alteration in decision making is one of my worst fears about alcohol, specifically alcohol and teenagers and young adults. The teenage brain is wired for addiction, the frontal lobes shut down in the early teens and this is the area that helps us make good decisions and not have what we like to call common sense. At the same time another part of the brain that acts on dopamine a chemical released when using alcohol or drugs is going at full speed ahead. This brain chemistry and working through these years is what leads to such high addictions in teenagers and young adults. Thankfully, the frontal lobes come back on line roughly in the mid to late twenties, and addiction potential then decreases.

What follows are my thoughts on the above, as well as recreational drugs. I mean to offend no one, and this comes from my experiences as a young adult and teenager who used alcohol as well as my experiences through practicing medicine both in the emergency room as well as in the clinic setting. If teenagers did not drink alcohol, they would be less likely to become pregnant. They would be less likely to rape and be raped. They would be less likely to get into car accidents. They would be less likely to shoot people. They would be less likely to abuse their loved ones physically as well as mentally, and they would be less likely to be abused themselves. They would be less likely to get arrested. They would be less likely to commit suicide. They would be more likely to graduate high school. They would be more likely to attend and complete college. They would be more likely to be physically fit. They would be more likely to marry of their choice under no undue influencing situation. Enough said. Extrapolate to all age groups.

# CHAPTER SEVEN

## Tobacco

I liked smoking. It calmed my nerves, it went along well with drinking. It was a social outlet to go smoke with others. It was the first thing I did in the morning and the last thing I did before bed. It went along with every meal. It went along with car rides. It was something I did everyday almost hourly for over five years. **Quitting it was one of the hardest things I have done in my life**. I tell you this, so you will appreciate that what follows is not from someone who has never smoked, it comes from someone who really liked to smoke but learned early on how bad it was for our bodies. I was in my early twenties, just figuring out that I could go to college and do something and learn things in life. I worked as an orderly in the operating room. I started noticing that some people did not wake up from anesthesia as well as others did, and it did not seem to be something age related. I would see young people wake up from anesthesia horribly and elderly people wake up easily and breathe easily. This made no sense to me. I finally asked one of the doctors one day what this pronounced difference was. Some people would wake up so well and others would not want to breathe at all and then when they finally did they would cough really violently. Turns out it was tobacco. It was a phenomenal difference. It is what showed me that I wanted nothing to do with it. It took these visuals over and over for me to be able to quit this drug. I will share with you later my success method as it has worked well for others. First, I will tell you a little of the statistics and realities of smoking and what it does to our body.

According to the Centers for Disease Control and Prevention (CDC), tobacco use remains the single largest preventable cause of death in the United States. In their most recent report-

- Over 480,000 deaths a year in our country are directly related to tobacco use. Just under ten percent of these deaths are actually from secondhand smoke. The majority of these deaths are from lung cancer, coronary heart disease and stroke.
- Healthcare dollars related to tobacco use amount to over $170,000,000,000 a year. Did you see all of those zeros? Incredible!

- $130,000,000,000 dollars are lost in work wages due to illnesses associated with tobacco.
- In 2014, 40 million Americans over 18 years of age reported smoking most days of their life.
- Overall mortality is three times higher in smokers than nonsmokers
- Life expectancy is ten years shorter for smokers
- One in five deaths in the US is due to smoking
- People who smoke are 23 times more likely to get lung cancer than non-smokers
- Middle aged men who smoke are four times more likely to have coronary heart disease than non-smokers

These statistics are real. As physicians, we see every day the consequences of smoking in premature deaths and diseases. In my practice, I really got quite tired of telling people all of the above reasons to quit smoking, I would talk and talk and talk some more and saw little result. I finally got to the point where I did not waste anymore of my time or my patients and I told them this simple truth. IF YOU DO NOT QUIT SMOKING, YOU WILL EITHER LIKELY DIE OF LUNG CANCER OR EMPHYSEMA (COPD)-YOU WOULD BE LUCKY TO GET THE LUNG CANCER, IT IS A MUCH SHORTER LESS PAINFUL DEATH THAN LIVING

WITH COPD AND BEING ON OXYGEN THE
LAST 15 YEARS OF YOUR LIFE.

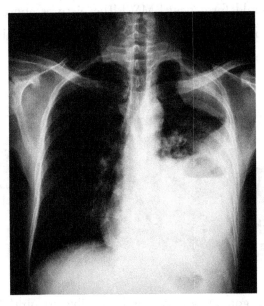

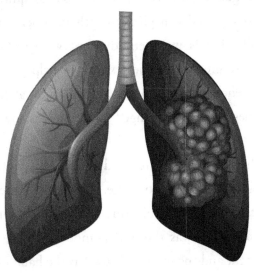

And what are you doing to get these premature death causing illnesses? You are paying more every month than you would for a new BMW! The pictures above show what lung cancer looks like. It is an unfortunately very common occurrence among lifelong smokers.

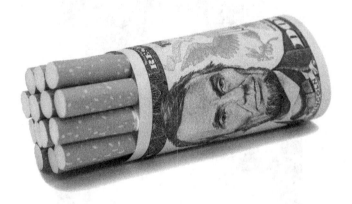

The good news, is – it is possible to quit! Many have done it and can give strength to others to do it. The following is my method from twenty plus years ago before great medicines existed to help you quit. I strongly encourage you to talk to your doctor about these medicines they have changed the lives of many for the better.

When I smoked, I realized there were two aspects of smoking that I had to battle. The first was the actual chemical addiction to nicotine and other chemicals in cigarettes. That was the easy component. The second component and the more difficult was the habit of doing it every day almost hourly. I came up with a plan to battle both of these aspects. For the chemical addiction, I realized I just needed to replace the tobacco and nicotine and taper it down. Over a two week period, I bought several cans of chewing tobacco in little pre wrapped individual pouches. I started with having four pouches a day and tapered it down by a pouch every couple days and over two weeks tapered to nothing. It didn't cost much and it worked. Chewing tobacco was disgusting to me and I knew it would ruin those pearly white teeth just like smoking so thankfully it didn't stick as a habit!

The behavioral component was much more difficult. I did two things to combat this. The first was I recognized specific times of the day that were especially related to smoking for me and I made a point to have something else I could put in my hand to play with instead of a cigarette. For me, one of the hardest times was in the car. I really liked to smoke when I drove in the car. So instead of a cigarette in my hand I had a couple of surgical forceps kind of like you use to take hooks out of a fish's mouth and in my car, I was always clicking and unclicking and twirling and playing with these little instruments instead of a cigarette. The second aspect of this was that I bought a pack of clove cigarettes. These things taste really good on the lips, but when you inhale them you think you might die. They hurt the lungs pretty badly. So when

I got to the point that I was sure I would die if I didn't have a cigarette, I would smoke and completely inhale one of these cloves. It usually made me sick in addition to hurting and so it lasted for one pack. That was my method of quitting. Some other suggestions for patients I have to occupy their minds and hands are to take up quilting, crocheting, fly tying, beadwork, jewelry making, in all honesty it really doesn't matter it is just something to do with your hands to replace smoking. It helps the mind get over the habit. Please talk to your doctor about medicines that are available now that can also help you quit. It is worth it.

# CHAPTER EIGHT

## What you should know about your doctor

Your doctor has ulterior motives. No harm is meant, in fact, quite the opposite. Most good doctors will try and talk you into doing some screening tests when you talk to them, or talk you into lifestyle choices that they know will help you. The basis of this is that we know if we catch diseases early on, there are much better, easier treatments for them. And even better, if we can make lifestyle changes early on, we can prevent a lot of disease and illness altogether. You know, the old saying "an ounce of prevention is worth a pound of cure" is really true….. It is much better to find out about your high blood pressure or cholesterol or diabetes and get them treated than have the heart attack that may kill you 5-10 years later because of these conditions not being treated. It is even that much better to change lifestyle habits and never get the illness or condition in the first place.

This is the job of the physician, to try and share with you things that we know to be true. Some physicians are better at the way they do this than others. Some offend. Some ridicule. But I believe all have the right intentions at heart. We want to help you. Give us the chance.

Printed in the United States
By Bookmasters